The 100-Year Life: A Blueprint for Longevity and Vitality

Introduction: The Search for a Century of Life

What if you could live to be 100? Not just surviving but thriving — enjoying the fullness of life, surrounded by loved ones, mentally sharp, physically agile, and spiritually fulfilled. What would that life look like? And more importantly, what would it take to get there?

In a world where technological advances are pushing the boundaries of human health and longevity, we find ourselves in an unprecedented era. Centenarians — those who live to 100 or beyond — are no longer anomalies. They are part of a growing global population that challenges our traditional understanding of aging. But the question remains: what is it that allows some people to live so long while others falter?

I've asked myself this question many times. As I watched family members and friends age, I became acutely aware of how varied our later years can be. Some people seem to retain a vitality that defies their chronological age, while others appear to wither under the weight of their years. The stark contrast fascinated me, and I knew I had to dig deeper.

This curiosity led me on a journey — a journey to understand what it truly means to live a long and meaningful life. I delved into the science of aging, but more than that, I explored the world's Blue Zones, where the highest concentrations of centenarians live. These communities in places like Okinawa, Sardinia, and Nicoya hold the secrets to longevity, and their way of life stands in sharp contrast to the fast-paced, stress-laden existence many of us lead today.

What struck me most in my research wasn't just the absence of disease or the presence of some mystical superfood. It was the simplicity of their lives. It was the way they connected with their families, the joy they found in daily movement, and the importance they placed on eating wholesome, plant-based meals. It was the meaning they derived from being part of something bigger than themselves — a purpose that carried them through their days, even in the face of adversity.

In this book, I want to take you through the lessons I've learned, weaving together scientific research, real-life stories from centenarians, and practical strategies that you can integrate into your own life. Living to 100 isn't just about adding years to your life — it's about adding life to your years. It's about making the choices today that will allow you to wake up, years from now, still feeling vibrant and engaged with the world around you.

So, what does it take to live to 100? It starts with understanding the factors that contribute to longevity and health. It's about taking control of your diet, movement, social connections, and mental well-being. It's about embracing the power of purpose and learning how to manage stress effectively. And it's about looking to the people who've already walked this path, taking inspiration from their wisdom and habits.

Are you ready to embark on this journey? Let's dive in.

Chapter 1: The Science of Longevity

When we think about living to 100, it's tempting to assume that genetics play the leading role. After all, some people seem "born lucky" — destined to live longer simply because of their family history. But the reality is far more nuanced. While genetics certainly have an influence, they account for only about 20–30% of a person's lifespan. The remaining 70–80%? That's determined by lifestyle choices — the foods we eat, the amount we move, the social connections we nurture, and the way we handle stress.

The Biology of Aging

To understand how we can live longer, it's essential to first grasp the biological processes that govern aging. Aging, at its core, is a gradual decline in the body's ability to repair itself. As we age, our cells accumulate damage, our immune systems weaken, and our DNA becomes more susceptible to mutations. Over time, these small, seemingly insignificant changes add up, leading to age-related diseases like cancer, cardiovascular issues, and cognitive decline.

One of the key drivers of aging is **oxidative stress** — a process that occurs when free radicals (unstable molecules that are byproducts of metabolism) damage our cells. Antioxidants, found in many fruits and vegetables, help neutralize these free radicals, which is why a diet rich in plant-based foods is so crucial for longevity. But oxidative stress is only one part of the puzzle. **Chronic inflammation** — often caused by poor diet, stress, and inactivity — also accelerates aging by damaging tissues and organs over time.

Another important aspect is **cellular regeneration**. Our bodies are constantly renewing themselves through the division of cells. However, each time a cell divides, the protective caps on the ends of our chromosomes, called **telomeres**, shorten. Eventually, telomeres become too short for the cell to divide safely, leading to cell death. Scientists have found that lifestyle factors, including diet, exercise, and stress management, can actually help slow down the rate of telomere shortening.

Finally, there's the issue of **insulin sensitivity**. As we age, our bodies often become less sensitive to insulin, leading to higher blood sugar levels and increased risk of type 2 diabetes. Diets rich in refined sugars and processed foods exacerbate this problem, while whole, plant-based foods improve insulin sensitivity and help regulate blood sugar levels.

Lessons from Blue Zones: The Role of Lifestyle in Aging

In studying the world's Blue Zones — regions where people regularly live to 100 — researchers have found striking similarities in their lifestyles. While these communities are spread across the globe and have unique cultures, the core principles they follow are remarkably consistent.

1. **Plant-Based Diets**: In every Blue Zone, the diet is predominantly plant-based. While some regions consume small amounts of animal products, the bulk of their meals come from beans, vegetables, and whole grains. In Okinawa, for example, sweet potatoes, tofu, and leafy greens are staples. In Sardinia, people enjoy a diet rich in whole grains, beans, and olive oil.

2. **Moderate Caloric Intake**: Centenarians tend to practice natural portion control, eating until they are about 80% full. The Okinawans have a phrase for this: *Hara hachi bu*. This practice prevents overeating and allows the body to function without the stress of excess calories.

3. **Daily Physical Activity**: People in Blue Zones don't typically engage in intense, structured exercise. Instead, they incorporate movement into their daily routines. They walk, garden, and do manual labor well into their old age. In Sardinia, it's common to see 90-year-olds still tending to their flocks or hiking mountainous terrain.

4. **Strong Social Networks**: Social connection is one of the most important, yet often overlooked, factors in longevity. Blue Zone communities are tightly knit, and people remain deeply connected with family and friends throughout their lives. This sense of belonging and support has profound effects on both mental and physical health.

5. **Purpose**: A sense of purpose is deeply embedded in Blue Zone cultures. In Okinawa, it's called *Ikigai*, which translates to "reason for being." In Costa Rica, it's referred to as *Plan de Vida* — a plan for life. Centenarians in these regions wake up each day with a clear sense of purpose, whether that's taking care of their family, contributing to their community, or engaging in a meaningful hobby.

Modern Science and Longevity

While the wisdom of Blue Zones provides a powerful blueprint for living longer, modern science has also made significant strides in understanding aging. **Caloric restriction** has emerged as one of the most promising avenues for increasing lifespan. Studies on animals have shown that reducing caloric intake by 20–30% can significantly extend lifespan and delay the onset of age-related diseases. This is thought to work by reducing oxidative stress and improving metabolic efficiency.

Intermittent fasting is another modern strategy that aligns with the eating patterns found in Blue Zones. Many centenarians naturally follow a form of intermittent fasting, either by limiting food intake to certain hours of the day or by having long breaks between meals. This practice helps to optimize metabolic function and promote cellular repair.

There is also growing interest in **anti-aging therapies** like gene editing and stem cell research. While these are exciting areas of development, they are still in the early stages and should be viewed as complementary, not primary, strategies for longevity.

Your First Steps Toward Longevity

The good news is that living to 100 isn't just about luck or genetics. By making simple, intentional choices each day, you can significantly influence your health and longevity. Start by looking at the key factors outlined in this chapter: adopt a more plant-based diet, incorporate daily movement, nurture meaningful social connections, and find your purpose. These changes may seem small, but over time, they can have a profound impact on your life.

As we continue in this book, we'll dive deeper into each of these topics, exploring how you can implement these strategies into your own life, no matter where you are on your journey. Remember, living to 100 is not about seeking perfection — it's about creating a life that's rich with meaning, connection, and vitality.

In the next chapter, we'll take a closer look at the specific foods that have helped people in Blue Zones achieve extraordinary lifespans. You'll discover how the right nutrition can transform your health and pave the way for a longer, more vibrant life.

Chapter 2: The Power of Nutrition: Eating for Longevity

Introduction: Food as Medicine

Food, in its purest form, has the power to heal, nourish, and extend life. But for many, the daily diet has become a battleground filled with processed, nutrient-poor, calorie-dense options. For those in the world's Blue Zones, food isn't just fuel — it's medicine, tradition, and community. This chapter will take a deep dive into the specific dietary patterns that have contributed to extraordinary longevity and explore how you can apply these principles to your own life.

The Foundation of Longevity: Plant-Based Diets

In Blue Zones, meals are centered around plant-based foods. Beans, vegetables, whole grains, nuts, and seeds form the cornerstone of their diet, while animal products play a minor role, if any. Let's explore the primary components of these diets, breaking them down by food groups, their nutrient profiles, and how they contribute to overall longevity.

1. Legumes: The Protein Powerhouse

- **Research on longevity and legumes:** Studies have shown that a diet rich in beans and lentils can reduce the risk of heart disease, cancer, and diabetes.
- **Types of legumes consumed in Blue Zones:** In Nicoya, black beans are a staple. In Okinawa, soybeans are the star. In Sardinia, chickpeas and fava beans feature prominently.
- **Practical ways to include more legumes in your diet:** Cooking techniques, recipes, and easy swaps for meat-based meals.

2. Leafy Greens: Nutrient Density Overload

- **Nutritional profile of greens:** Explore the vitamin and mineral density of dark leafy greens like kale, spinach, collard greens, and wild herbs.
- **The role of greens in preventing disease:** Studies show that regular consumption of greens lowers the risk of cognitive decline and chronic disease.
- **Stories from centenarians:** Real-life examples from Blue Zones where daily consumption of greens is a non-negotiable habit.
- **Easy integration into modern life:** Smoothies, salads, soups, and sautées.

3. Whole Grains: Ancient Carbohydrates

- **The Sardinian diet and whole grains:** Sardinians consume traditional whole grains like barley and farro. This section explores their historical context, how they're prepared, and their health benefits.
- **Modern grains vs. ancient grains:** The contrast between refined grains and the nutrient-rich whole grains of the past.
- **Practical tips for adding whole grains:** Recipes and ideas for incorporating farro, bulgur, quinoa, and more into your meals.

The Science Behind the Blue Zone Diet

1. Caloric Restriction: Less is More

- **Hara Hachi Bu:** The Okinawan practice of eating until 80% full and its impact on caloric restriction, metabolic health, and aging.
- **The science of caloric restriction:** Studies in animal models and humans that show how limiting caloric intake without malnutrition can slow aging processes.
- **How to implement caloric restriction mindfully:** Practical tips for slowing down eating, savoring food, and recognizing satiety signals.

2. The Role of Fasting: Cellular Regeneration

- **Intermittent fasting in Blue Zones:** Exploring how natural patterns of fasting (skipping meals, longer breaks between dinner and breakfast) mirror current trends in intermittent fasting.
- **The science of fasting and longevity:** How fasting triggers autophagy, the body's process of cleaning out damaged cells and regenerating new ones.
- **Simple fasting strategies:** Time-restricted eating, periodic fasting, and how to safely introduce fasting into your life.

Beyond the Plate: How Food and Community Interact

Food is never consumed in isolation in Blue Zones. It's a communal activity, a time to connect, share stories, and laugh. This section will explore the **rituals around meals** in Blue Zones and how communal eating plays a critical role in mental and emotional well-being, which directly influences longevity.

1. The Importance of Rituals Around Meals

- **Meals as social glue:** In Sardinia, families gather daily for communal meals. In Okinawa, the elderly share meals with younger generations. How these rituals reinforce a sense of belonging.
- **Storytelling and food:** How sharing food and stories creates a bond that sustains communities across generations.

2. Slowing Down and Savoring

- **The mindful eating practices in Blue Zones:** How slow food movements and mindful eating contribute to better digestion, lower stress, and stronger social connections.
- **Practical mindfulness techniques:** Strategies for incorporating mindful eating into busy modern lives, from savoring the first bite to putting down your fork between bites.

Conclusion: Food as a Lifelong Prescription

Nutrition for longevity isn't about following a strict diet or depriving yourself. It's about developing a sustainable, joyful relationship with food that supports health, community, and purpose. By following the dietary principles laid out in this chapter — focusing on plant-based foods, mindful eating, and occasional caloric restriction — you'll not only add years to your life but also life to your years.

Chapter 3: The Power of Movement: Staying Active for Life

Introduction: Movement as a Way of Life

The gym culture that dominates much of the Western world is virtually nonexistent in Blue Zones. Centenarians don't "exercise" in the way many of us do — but they are constantly moving. Their lives are full of low-intensity, natural movements that keep their bodies agile and strong well into old age. In this chapter, we'll explore the role of daily movement, the benefits of low-impact activity, and how you can bring more natural movement into your life.

Movement Patterns in Blue Zones

1. Daily Activity in Okinawa

- **The role of gardening:** Gardening is a common activity in Okinawa, where elders spend hours tending to their crops. This isn't just exercise; it's a way to stay connected to nature and cultivate a sense of purpose.
- **Sitting on the floor:** Okinawans sit and rise from the floor multiple times a day, which contributes to their leg strength and balance — factors critical to longevity.
- **The science of low-impact, high-frequency movement:** Research shows that constant low-intensity movement is more beneficial for longevity than brief bouts of intense exercise. Explore the effects on cardiovascular health, joint function, and mental health.

2. The Shepherds of Sardinia: Walking as a Lifelong Habit

- **Sardinian shepherds and mountain living:** The rugged terrain of Sardinia requires constant walking, and this daily movement is part of what keeps these shepherds healthy into their 90s and beyond.
- **The physiological benefits of walking:** Studies show that walking can lower blood pressure, improve mental clarity, and enhance mood.
- **Practical ways to add walking into modern life:** Whether it's walking meetings, taking the stairs, or getting off the bus a stop early, this section will offer strategies to incorporate walking into daily routines.

3. Nicoya's Manual Labor: Strength in Simplicity

- **The value of manual labor:** In Nicoya, many centenarians continue to work with their hands well into old age. Whether it's chopping wood or repairing tools, these activities keep muscles strong and minds sharp.
- **The link between strength training and longevity:** Explore the science behind muscle mass, strength, and their critical roles in preventing falls and maintaining independence in old age.

Structured Exercise vs. Natural Movement

In modern society, we tend to compartmentalize movement into "exercise" and "everything else." But in Blue Zones, exercise is a part of everyday life — it's functional, purposeful, and integrated into daily routines.

1. Why Less Is More: The Case Against High-Intensity Workouts

- **The hidden risks of intense exercise:** Explore how high-intensity, high-impact exercise can lead to burnout, injury, and stress when overdone.
- **The benefits of natural, moderate-intensity movement:** How activities like gardening, walking, and household chores mimic the movements that promote longevity.

2. Building a Life of Movement Without a Gym

- **Creative ways to incorporate movement:** From walking instead of driving to using a standing desk, explore how to integrate more movement into your day.
- **Micro-workouts for busy people:** Short, practical exercises you can do throughout the day to keep your body in motion.
- **The power of stretching and flexibility:** Why maintaining flexibility is key to aging gracefully and how simple stretches can make a big impact.

Mental Health and Movement

Physical activity isn't just good for the body — it's essential for the brain. Movement promotes the release of endorphins, lowers stress levels, and has been shown to protect against cognitive decline.

1. The Cognitive Benefits of Regular Activity

- **Exercise and neuroplasticity:** How physical activity encourages the brain to form new connections, helping to preserve cognitive function as we age.
- **Case studies from Blue Zones:** Stories of centenarians who stay mentally sharp through regular movement, whether it's by walking, gardening, or manual labor.

2. Movement as a Stress Reliever

- **The link between stress and aging:** Chronic stress accelerates aging by increasing inflammation, damaging cells, and shortening telomeres.

Movement, especially low-intensity, stress-relieving activities like yoga or walking, can help reverse this damage.

- **Mind-body exercises:** Yoga, tai chi, and qi gong as tools for longevity. Practical tips for incorporating these mind-body practices into your routine.

Conclusion: Movement as Medicine

Longevity isn't about punishing yourself in the gym or running marathons. It's about making movement a joyful, natural part of your life. Whether you're walking, gardening, or doing simple stretches at home, staying active keeps your body resilient, your mind sharp, and your spirit vibrant. By incorporating these lessons from the Blue Zones, you can create a lifestyle of movement that sustains you for the long haul.

Chapter 4: Stress Reduction and Mindfulness: Living with Purpose and Peace

Introduction: The Impact of Stress on Longevity

Stress is an unavoidable part of life, but how we manage it can determine how well we age. Chronic stress has been linked to numerous health issues, from heart disease to cognitive decline. In Blue Zones, stress is managed through a combination of lifestyle, mindset, and cultural rituals that foster relaxation, community, and purpose. This chapter will explore how reducing stress and fostering mindfulness can add years to your life and quality to those years.

The Effects of Chronic Stress on the Body

1. How Stress Ages Us

- **The science of stress and aging:** Chronic stress shortens telomeres, the protective caps at the ends of our DNA strands, which leads to premature aging.
- **Inflammation and disease:** Stress increases inflammation, which is a major driver of diseases like cancer, Alzheimer's, and heart disease.
- **Case studies of stress-free centenarians:** Stories from Blue Zones where low-stress living is the norm and its correlation with long, healthy lives.

2. The Stress-Longevity Paradox

- **Why high-achievers may not live as long:** The link between stress, success, and early death — and what high-performing individuals can learn from Blue Zones about slowing down.
- **The science of relaxation:** Studies showing how regular relaxation practices can reverse some of the damage caused by chronic stress.

Stress-Relief Rituals from Blue Zones

In Blue Zones, daily life naturally incorporates stress-relieving rituals. These aren't necessarily formal practices like meditation or yoga, but simple habits that encourage relaxation, connection, and mindfulness.

1. Sardinia's Siesta: The Power of Rest

- **The science behind naps:** Research shows that short naps during the day can lower blood pressure, reduce stress, and boost cognitive function.

- **Creating a daily rest ritual:** How to carve out time for rest in your day, even if it's just 20 minutes of quiet time.
- **Resting without guilt:** How to overcome the societal pressure to constantly be productive and the importance of rest for longevity.

2. Okinawa's Ikigai: Living with Purpose

- **What is ikigai?:** The Okinawan concept of "a reason for being" is central to their long lives. We'll explore how having a sense of purpose can keep you mentally and physically active, well into your later years.
- **The psychological and physical benefits of purpose:** How having a sense of purpose reduces stress, increases resilience, and even boosts immunity.
- **How to find your ikigai:** Practical tips for identifying what gives your life meaning and how to incorporate it into your daily routine.

3. Nicoya's Pura Vida: Embracing a Positive Mindset

- **The philosophy of "Pura Vida":** In Costa Rica, the Nicoyans live by the phrase "Pura Vida" or "pure life," a reminder to live simply, stress less, and enjoy life's small moments.
- **The health benefits of a positive mindset:** Research shows that optimism and positive thinking are linked to longer lifespans and better health outcomes.
- **How to cultivate positivity:** Practical exercises to reframe negative thoughts, focus on gratitude, and bring more joy into your life.

Mindfulness for Longevity

Mindfulness — the practice of being present in the moment — has been shown to reduce stress, improve emotional regulation, and enhance overall well-being. In Blue Zones, mindfulness isn't a formal practice but a natural part of daily life.

1. Mindfulness and the Aging Brain

- **The neurobiology of mindfulness:** How mindfulness practices increase gray matter, improve focus, and delay cognitive decline.
- **Case studies of mindfulness in Blue Zones:** How daily tasks like gardening, cooking, or walking can be transformed into mindful, stress-relieving activities.

2. Simple Mindfulness Practices for Daily Life

- **Breathwork for relaxation:** Simple breathing exercises that can lower stress in minutes.

- **Mindful eating:** How to use your meals as an opportunity for mindfulness, savoring each bite, and reducing stress at the table.
- **Mindful movement:** Walking, yoga, and stretching as opportunities for mindfulness.

Conclusion: Cultivating Peace in a Busy World

Stress will always be a part of life, but how we manage it determines its impact on our health and longevity. By adopting the stress-relieving practices of the world's longest-living people, you can cultivate a life of purpose, peace, and mindfulness. In doing so, you'll not only reduce your risk of disease but also add joy and meaning to your years.

Chapter 5: The Social Connection: Building Strong Relationships for Longevity

Introduction: The Power of Relationships

Human beings are inherently social creatures, and our need for connection runs deep. As much as a healthy diet and regular movement are important for longevity, strong, positive relationships may be just as critical, if not more. In fact, research consistently shows that people with strong social ties live longer, healthier lives. In the Blue Zones, social connection is deeply embedded into everyday life. Whether through family, friends, or community, people in these regions foster relationships that help them thrive well into their 90s and beyond.

This chapter will explore the profound connection between social bonds and longevity, drawing insights from the world's longest-living populations. We'll delve into why relationships are essential for health, how they impact physical and mental well-being, and how to cultivate and sustain meaningful relationships that add years to your life.

The Health Benefits of Strong Social Connections

1. Reduced Stress and Better Emotional Health

- **The buffering effect of relationships:** One of the primary reasons social connections improve longevity is their ability to buffer against stress. When life gets difficult, having someone to talk to, lean on, or confide in reduces the emotional burden.
- **How stress shortens lifespans:** Chronic stress can lead to inflammation, hormonal imbalances, and premature aging. Studies show that people with strong social support are less likely to experience these harmful effects.
- **Oxytocin and bonding:** When we form close connections with others, our bodies release oxytocin, the "bonding hormone." Oxytocin helps calm our stress response, reduces blood pressure, and fosters a sense of well-being.

2. Loneliness and Its Detrimental Effects on Health

- **The loneliness epidemic:** In modern societies, despite the proliferation of technology and social media, more people report feeling isolated than ever before. Loneliness has been linked to a host of health problems, including heart disease, depression, and even early death.

- **Comparing loneliness with smoking:** Research from Brigham Young University found that loneliness can have the same detrimental effect on health as smoking 15 cigarettes a day.
- **Case studies from Blue Zones:** In places like Okinawa, people rarely live alone. Older individuals are integrated into the fabric of the community and never feel isolated. This sense of belonging plays a major role in their longevity.

3. Better Physical Health Through Social Bonds

- **Heart health and community:** Studies show that people who are more socially connected have better cardiovascular health. They're less likely to suffer from high blood pressure, heart disease, or strokes.
- **The role of social support in recovery:** People with strong support systems recover faster from illnesses or surgeries, as they often have someone encouraging them to adhere to medical advice or accompany them to appointments.

Social Structures in Blue Zones: What We Can Learn

In each of the Blue Zones, strong social networks play an essential role in the daily lives of centenarians. Relationships are prioritized over material success, and people often spend a significant amount of time with loved ones.

1. Okinawa: Moai Groups

- **What is a Moai?:** In Okinawa, people belong to lifelong social networks called "moais." These groups provide financial, emotional, and social support. Moai groups meet regularly, celebrate life's milestones together, and provide companionship through life's difficulties.
- **The health benefits of belonging to a Moai:** Research shows that people who belong to such close-knit groups live longer because they have constant emotional and social support.
- **Creating your own Moai:** You don't need to live in Okinawa to benefit from the concept of a Moai. This section will offer practical advice on how to form your own small, supportive social group.

2. Sardinia: Family First

- **Multigenerational households in Sardinia:** In Sardinia, it's common for families to live together or near one another. Grandparents are deeply involved in the lives of their grandchildren, creating a sense of purpose and responsibility for the older generation.
- **The impact of family support on longevity:** Sardinian centenarians attribute their long lives to the love and care they receive from their

families. They feel valued, respected, and important, which fosters a positive outlook and reduces stress.
- **How to strengthen family ties:** In the modern world, it's easy to become disconnected from family due to physical distance or busy lives. This section will explore ways to nurture and rebuild familial relationships for stronger social support.

3. Nicoya: Community and Faith

- **Pura Vida lifestyle:** The Costa Rican lifestyle is rooted in a sense of community, friendliness, and faith. Nicoyans frequently gather for community events, and they take care of one another in times of need.
- **The role of faith in longevity:** Belonging to a religious or spiritual community has been shown to improve longevity, likely due to the social networks and emotional resilience it provides. People in Nicoya often turn to their faith for comfort during difficult times, which lowers stress and provides a sense of peace.

Cultivating Meaningful Connections

You don't need to live in a Blue Zone to build meaningful relationships that will support your health and well-being. This section will explore practical strategies to develop and maintain close, supportive social bonds in today's fast-paced, often disconnected world.

1. Nurturing Existing Relationships

- **Making time for people:** In a busy world, it can be easy to neglect relationships. However, prioritizing time for friends and family is one of the most effective ways to maintain strong connections.
- **Improving communication:** Good communication is the foundation of any strong relationship. Learning how to express yourself clearly, listen actively, and resolve conflicts in a healthy way will strengthen your social bonds.

2. Building New Social Connections

- **Finding your tribe:** Whether through shared interests, community events, or professional organizations, finding like-minded people is key to building new friendships.
- **Getting involved in your community:** Volunteering, attending local events, or joining clubs are all ways to meet new people and foster a sense of belonging.

- **Overcoming social anxiety:** If building new relationships feels overwhelming, this section will provide strategies for overcoming social anxiety and taking small steps toward connection.

3. Staying Connected in a Digital World

- **The pros and cons of digital relationships:** While online connections can provide support and companionship, they shouldn't replace face-to-face interactions. This section will explore how to balance digital and real-world relationships.
- **Using technology to enhance relationships:** Practical tips for using technology to stay in touch with loved ones, even when distance separates you.

Conclusion: Relationships as the Key to Longevity

At the heart of living a long, fulfilling life is the quality of your relationships. Whether it's family, friends, or your community, these bonds give life meaning and provide the support we need to thrive. By nurturing and investing in your relationships, you'll not only improve your emotional and mental well-being but also add years to your life.

Chapter 6: Purpose and Passion: Living with Meaning for a Longer Life

Introduction: The Link Between Purpose and Longevity

Purpose is a powerful force that can drive us to live longer, healthier lives. Having a sense of purpose — whether it's found in work, hobbies, relationships, or spiritual practices — is a common thread in the lives of centenarians from the Blue Zones. These individuals wake up each day with a clear sense of what they need to do and why it matters, and this sense of direction gives their lives meaning.

In this chapter, we'll explore how having a strong sense of purpose is tied to longevity, how people in the Blue Zones define their purpose, and how you can discover and cultivate your own purpose to lead a more fulfilling, long life.

The Science of Purpose and Longevity

1. Ikigai: The Okinawan Concept of Purpose

- **What is Ikigai?:** In Okinawa, the term "ikigai" refers to one's reason for being. It's the thing that gets you out of bed in the morning — the intersection of what you love, what you're good at, what the world needs, and what you can be paid for.
- **The health benefits of ikigai:** Research shows that people with a strong sense of purpose live longer and experience lower rates of depression and anxiety. They're also more resilient in the face of challenges, which can help protect against the health effects of stress.
- **How to find your ikigai:** This section will provide practical exercises to help you identify your own ikigai by reflecting on your passions, skills, and values.

2. The Role of Purpose in Aging Well

- **Purpose and cognitive health:** Studies suggest that people who have a clear sense of purpose are less likely to experience cognitive decline as they age. Purpose stimulates the brain and keeps it engaged, which may protect against dementia and other age-related cognitive disorders.
- **Purpose and physical health:** People with a sense of purpose tend to take better care of themselves. They're more likely to stay active, eat healthily, and adhere to medical advice, all of which contribute to better overall health.

- **Purpose as a stress reliever:** Having a sense of purpose can also help mitigate the effects of stress, as it gives individuals a reason to persevere through difficult times.

How People in Blue Zones Live with Purpose

In Blue Zones, purpose isn't something people retire from. It's a lifelong pursuit that evolves over time. Whether it's taking care of family, engaging in meaningful work, or contributing to the community, centenarians in Blue Zones remain active and involved in purposeful activities well into their later years.

1. Purpose Through Family and Community in Sardinia

- **The role of family in Sardinian life:** In Sardinia, older adults often take on the role of caretakers for grandchildren or community elders. This gives them a sense of responsibility and purpose, knowing they are contributing to the well-being of others.
- **How purpose keeps Sardinian elders active:** Centenarians in Sardinia often attribute their longevity to staying active and involved in their community. Whether it's farming, cooking, or mentoring younger generations, their sense of purpose keeps them physically and mentally engaged.

2. Volunteering and Contribution in Nicoya

- **Giving back to the community:** In Nicoya, Costa Rica, older adults often spend their time volunteering or contributing to the community in meaningful ways. Whether through religious organizations, local groups, or helping neighbors, their sense of purpose comes from serving others.
- **The health benefits of giving back:** Research shows that volunteering and helping others can reduce the risk of depression, increase happiness, and even lower mortality rates. The act of giving back creates a sense of connection and meaning that sustains individuals through life's challenges.

Finding Your Own Purpose

You don't need to be a centenarian to find purpose and passion in your life. This section will guide you through practical exercises to help you discover and cultivate your sense of purpose, no matter where you are in life.

1. Reflecting on Your Values and Passions

- **What excites you?:** Start by reflecting on the activities, causes, or people that make you feel excited or energized. These can be clues to where your passions lie.
- **What are your core values?:** Identifying your values — what matters most to you in life — can help you determine what kind of purpose will be most fulfilling. Is it family, work, community, or spirituality?
- **Aligning purpose with values:** Once you've identified your values, consider how your daily life aligns with them. Are you spending time on what truly matters to you? If not, what changes can you make?

2. Setting Goals That Inspire You

- **Creating a sense of direction:** Purpose often comes from setting and working toward goals that matter to you. Whether it's starting a new hobby, deepening relationships, or contributing to a cause, setting meaningful goals can give your life focus and purpose.
- **Overcoming obstacles:** It's common to face obstacles or challenges on the path to purpose. This section will provide strategies for overcoming setbacks and staying motivated.

3. Finding Purpose in Every Season of Life

- **Purpose at every age:** Whether you're young and just starting out or older and looking for a new direction, it's never too late to discover your purpose. Purpose can evolve and change as you move through different stages of life.
- **Purpose in retirement:** Many people struggle with finding purpose after they retire, as they lose the structure and identity that work provides. This section will explore ways to redefine purpose in retirement through hobbies, volunteer work, and new opportunities.

Conclusion: Living with Purpose for a Longer, Happier Life

Living with purpose is one of the most powerful ways to add meaning and fulfillment to your life, and it's also a key factor in longevity. By discovering and nurturing your sense of purpose, you can stay active, engaged, and motivated well into your later years. Whether it's through family, work, community, or personal passions, finding your purpose is essential to living not just a long life, but a life full of joy and meaning.

Chapter 7: The Power of Movement: Staying Active for a Century

Introduction: Movement as a Lifelong Practice

In the journey to living a long and healthy life, staying active is non-negotiable. Movement doesn't have to mean intense workouts at the gym or rigorous sports. In fact, one of the key lessons from the world's Blue Zones is that centenarians don't have structured exercise routines, but they incorporate natural, daily movement into their lives. Whether it's walking to work, gardening, or simply moving around the home, physical activity is a way of life.

This chapter dives deep into how different forms of movement contribute to longevity, examining everything from low-intensity activities to the importance of muscle strength, flexibility, and cardiovascular health. We'll also explore the practical ways you can stay active throughout life, and how to make movement a joyful and natural part of your routine.

The Science Behind Physical Activity and Longevity

1. Movement and Cardiovascular Health

- **Heart health and longevity:** Cardiovascular disease is one of the leading causes of death, but regular physical activity is one of the most effective ways to reduce risk. Even moderate exercise like walking can dramatically improve heart health, lower blood pressure, and reduce the risk of heart attacks and strokes.
- **Examples from Blue Zones:** In Sardinia and Ikaria, daily movement through walking, farming, or manual labor keeps their cardiovascular systems strong. The natural landscapes often require walking up and down hills, providing incidental exercise that enhances endurance.

2. Strength and Balance for Aging Gracefully

- **Why muscle strength matters:** As we age, maintaining muscle mass is crucial for mobility, balance, and independence. Strength training or weight-bearing exercises help prevent falls, a leading cause of injury in older adults, and also boost metabolism.
- **Blue Zone activities that strengthen muscles:** Sardinian shepherds and Okinawan gardeners engage in physical labor that naturally builds strength. The lesson here is that it's not necessary to lift weights at a gym—everyday tasks like carrying groceries, squatting to garden, or moving furniture can serve the same purpose.

3. Flexibility and Joint Health for Mobility

- **The role of flexibility:** As we age, maintaining flexibility becomes critical for reducing stiffness, improving posture, and preventing injury. Yoga, tai chi, and simple stretching can keep joints supple and functional.
- **Blue Zone practices:** In Okinawa, many centenarians practice martial arts or gardening, both of which require flexibility and balance. Simple daily movements, such as squatting or bending, keep their bodies limber.

Movement Practices in Blue Zones

In Blue Zones, movement is an integral part of life. Here's how centenarians in these regions stay active:

1. Walking as a Way of Life

- **Okinawa and Nicoya:** Whether walking to visit a neighbor, walking to the market, or simply walking to enjoy the fresh air, this low-impact activity is a consistent habit for centenarians.
- **The benefits of walking:** Walking improves cardiovascular health, strengthens bones, and boosts mental well-being. Studies show that walking 30 minutes a day can lower the risk of premature death by up to 30%.

2. Gardening as Movement

- **Okinawan gardeners:** Gardening is one of the most common activities among Okinawan centenarians. The constant bending, pulling, and squatting involved in tending plants keep their bodies active and engaged.
- **The mental benefits of gardening:** In addition to physical exercise, gardening provides mental stimulation, reduces stress, and fosters a sense of purpose.

3. Manual Labor and Daily Chores

- **Sardinian farmers:** In Sardinia, many centenarians continue to engage in farming, herding sheep, or tending to livestock well into their 90s. These tasks are not only physically demanding but also provide purpose and connection to the land.
- **Housework and everyday movement:** From sweeping floors to chopping wood, household chores in the Blue Zones are a natural way to incorporate movement into daily life.

Incorporating Movement Into Your Life

It's never too late to start moving more. You don't need to adopt an intense exercise regimen to reap the benefits of movement. Instead, focus on integrating small, sustainable habits into your routine:

1. Daily Walking

- **Walk with purpose:** Make walking a part of your day by walking to run errands, walking after meals, or taking a morning stroll.
- **Walk with others:** Walking with friends or family not only helps you stay active but also fosters social connections.

2. Natural Movement in Daily Chores

- **Find opportunities to move:** Carry your groceries instead of using a cart, take the stairs instead of the elevator, or bike instead of driving.
- **Turn chores into exercise:** Yard work, cleaning, or rearranging furniture can all be ways to stay physically active while accomplishing necessary tasks.

3. Strength and Flexibility Practices

- **Bodyweight exercises:** Incorporate bodyweight exercises such as squats, lunges, or push-ups into your day. These exercises improve muscle strength without requiring equipment.
- **Stretching and mobility work:** Stretch daily to improve flexibility and reduce tension in muscles and joints. Practices like yoga or tai chi can also help build strength, balance, and flexibility.

Conclusion: Movement as Medicine

The lesson from the world's longest-living people is clear: movement is medicine. By integrating natural, low-impact movement into daily life, you can significantly improve your health, increase your longevity, and enhance your quality of life. The key is not extreme exercise but consistent, mindful movement that brings joy and purpose to your day.

Chapter 8: Rest and Recovery: The Importance of Sleep and Relaxation

Introduction: Sleep and Longevity

In the quest for longevity, one of the most overlooked factors is rest, especially quality sleep. We often think of sleep as a passive activity, but in reality, it's during sleep that the body repairs, rejuvenates, and restores itself. Centenarians in Blue Zones prioritize rest, ensuring that their bodies get the recovery they need to stay healthy, vibrant, and resilient into old age.

This chapter will explore the critical role of sleep and relaxation in promoting longevity. We'll look at the science behind sleep, the benefits of napping, and the practices of centenarians who incorporate rest into their lives.

The Science of Sleep: Why It Matters

1. Sleep and Physical Health

- **Healing and regeneration during sleep:** During sleep, the body repairs muscles, restores energy, and regulates hormones. Growth hormones are released, tissues are repaired, and immune function is enhanced.
- **Sleep and longevity:** Studies show that adults who regularly get between seven to nine hours of sleep per night tend to live longer than those who are chronically sleep-deprived.

2. Sleep and Cognitive Function

- **Brain health and memory:** Sleep is essential for brain function. It helps consolidate memories, clear waste products from brain cells, and supports cognitive function. Poor sleep has been linked to an increased risk of dementia and Alzheimer's disease.
- **Mental clarity and decision-making:** Getting enough sleep improves concentration, focus, and decision-making, all of which contribute to a healthier, longer life.

Rest Practices in Blue Zones

Centenarians in Blue Zones understand the value of rest and recovery. Here's how they incorporate it into their daily routines:

1. Okinawa: Napping and Restorative Practices

- **Midday napping:** Many Okinawans practice napping as part of their daily routine. A short nap in the middle of the day allows the body to recharge, reduce stress, and boost cognitive function.
- **Mindfulness and relaxation:** In addition to napping, Okinawans often practice mindfulness or spend time in nature, which helps reduce stress and promote relaxation.

2. Ikaria: The Mediterranean Siesta

- **The culture of the siesta:** In Ikaria, Greece, taking a midday rest is a normal part of daily life. The traditional siesta, lasting between 30 minutes and an hour, helps reduce stress, lowers the risk of heart disease, and promotes longevity.
- **Slow living and relaxation:** The Ikarian way of life is focused on slow living. People in Ikaria take their time with meals, socializing, and daily tasks, reducing the stress that can come with rushing through life.

3. Sardinia: The Importance of Leisure

- **Rest after labor:** Sardinians often engage in manual labor, but they also value leisure and relaxation. After a morning of work, it's common to spend the afternoon resting or socializing with family and friends.
- **Social relaxation:** Spending time with loved ones is a form of relaxation in Sardinia. The connection with others helps reduce stress and create a sense of emotional well-being.

Practical Tips for Better Sleep and Rest

In today's fast-paced world, getting enough rest can be a challenge. Here are practical ways to prioritize sleep and relaxation:

1. Create a Relaxing Sleep Environment

- **Optimize your bedroom:** Make your bedroom a sanctuary for sleep by minimizing noise, keeping the room cool, and eliminating bright lights.
- **Bedtime routine:** Develop a bedtime routine that signals to your body that it's time to sleep. This could include reading, gentle stretching, or meditation.

2. Take Breaks During the Day

- **Power naps:** Short naps of 20 to 30 minutes during the day can recharge your energy and improve mental clarity without interfering with nighttime sleep.

- **Mindful breaks:** Take short breaks during your workday to stretch, breathe deeply, or step outside for fresh air. These breaks can reduce stress and prevent burnout.

3. Prioritize Relaxation and Leisure

- **Incorporate downtime into your day:** Whether it's reading, gardening, or simply sitting in silence, find moments of peace and relaxation throughout your day.
- **Disconnect from screens:** Limit screen time, especially before bed, as blue light from phones and computers can interfere with your body's natural sleep cycle.

Conclusion: The Art of Rest for a Long Life

In the pursuit of longevity, rest and relaxation are just as important as diet and exercise. By prioritizing sleep and taking time to relax, you can reduce stress, improve mental and physical health, and increase your chances of living a long, healthy life. The world's centenarians show us that it's not just about working hard, but also about knowing when to rest.

Chapter 9: Connection and Community: The Social Factor in Longevity

Introduction: The Importance of Social Bonds

Human beings are inherently social creatures. Our need for connection and community goes beyond just friendship and companionship—it's deeply tied to our overall health and well-being. Studies show that strong social relationships can lower the risk of premature death, reduce the likelihood of developing chronic illnesses, and even improve mental health.

In this chapter, we'll explore the power of social connections in promoting longevity, drawing insights from Blue Zones where community is central to daily life. We'll look at how social bonds support physical and mental health, and offer strategies to build and maintain meaningful relationships throughout your life.

Social Connections and Longevity: What the Research Says

1. The Link Between Loneliness and Poor Health

- **Loneliness and early death:** Chronic loneliness is a significant predictor of early death. It has been linked to an increased risk of heart disease, stroke, depression, and even dementia. In contrast, people with strong social ties tend to live longer, healthier lives.
- **Social isolation and inflammation:** Studies show that social isolation can increase inflammation in the body, contributing to a host of chronic diseases. In contrast, strong social bonds help regulate the immune system and reduce harmful inflammation.

2. The Role of Relationships in Mental Health

- **Social support and emotional well-being:** Having a strong network of family, friends, and community members can act as a buffer against stress, anxiety, and depression. These relationships provide emotional support during difficult times and enhance feelings of happiness and purpose.

- **Building resilience through connection:** Social connections promote resilience, helping people bounce back from adversity and stay mentally strong. This resilience is crucial for maintaining health and vitality into old age.

Community and Connection in Blue Zones

The longest-living people in Blue Zones often have deep-rooted social networks that provide them with emotional, practical, and sometimes even physical support. Here's how they cultivate strong community bonds:

1. Okinawa: The Power of the Moai

- **What is a moai?:** In Okinawa, people form lifelong social groups called moais. These groups meet regularly to offer emotional and financial support to one another. The bond within a moai is so strong that members often look after each other as they age, providing a powerful sense of community and belonging.
- **How moais promote longevity:** The close-knit relationships within a moai reduce stress, provide a sense of purpose, and create a safety net for members, all of which contribute to their long, healthy lives.

2. Sardinia: Multi-generational Living

- **Families staying close:** In Sardinia, it's common for multiple generations to live together or near one another. This proximity creates a strong sense of community, where elders are respected and supported, and family bonds are strengthened.
- **The benefits of multi-generational living:** Living with or near family members not only fosters close relationships but also provides emotional support and helps share the burdens of daily life. Elders in these families often take care of grandchildren, which keeps them active and engaged.

3. Nicoya: A Deep Sense of Faith and Community

- **Faith and social bonds:** In Nicoya, Costa Rica, centenarians often attribute their longevity to their faith and strong community ties. Religion plays a central role in their lives, providing them with a sense of purpose and belonging.
- **Religious gatherings and social connection:** Regular religious gatherings offer an opportunity to socialize and strengthen community bonds, which in turn promote emotional well-being and reduce feelings of isolation.

Strengthening Your Own Social Connections

No matter where you are in life, it's never too late to build and strengthen your social network. Here are some ways to foster meaningful relationships:

1. Investing in Close Relationships

- **Quality over quantity:** It's not about having a large number of friends, but rather cultivating a few deep, meaningful relationships. Invest time and energy into the relationships that matter most to you, whether it's family, friends, or a partner.
- **Expressing gratitude and appreciation:** Regularly expressing gratitude and appreciation to those close to you strengthens bonds and creates a deeper sense of connection.

2. Joining Groups and Communities

- **Finding like-minded people:** Join groups, clubs, or organizations that align with your interests, values, or hobbies. Whether it's a book club, a religious group, or a fitness class, being part of a community can enhance your sense of belonging.
- **Volunteering and giving back:** Volunteering is a great way to meet new people and give back to the community. It provides a sense of purpose and can lead to strong social connections.

3. Maintaining Relationships Over Time

- **Staying in touch:** Maintaining long-term friendships takes effort. Regularly check in with friends, call or visit family members, and show up for important events. Even small gestures, like a text or a phone call, can help keep connections strong.
- **Navigating conflict:** Conflict is a natural part of relationships. Learn to navigate disagreements with grace, listening actively and seeking solutions that honor both parties.

Conclusion: Connection as a Key to Longevity

The science is clear: social connections are essential for a long, healthy life. By investing in your relationships and building a strong community, you not only improve your emotional and mental health, but you also increase your chances of living a longer, more fulfilling life. The wisdom of the world's centenarians shows us that connection and community are just as important as diet and exercise in the pursuit of longevity.

Conclusion: The Path to 100 Years and Beyond

As we've explored throughout this book, the path to a long, healthy life is not about radical changes or extreme diets. It's about incorporating simple, sustainable habits that promote physical, mental, and emotional well-being. From the lessons of the world's longest-living people in Blue Zones to the latest research on nutrition, movement, sleep, and social connection, the keys to longevity are within your reach.

Key Takeaways

1. **Eat for Health and Longevity**: Focus on whole, plant-based foods, and enjoy meals with family and friends. Prioritize local, seasonal foods that nourish both body and soul.

2. **Stay Active, Naturally**: Incorporate movement into your daily life, whether through walking, gardening, or housework. Remember, it's not about intense exercise but about consistent, natural movement.

3. **Rest and Recover**: Prioritize sleep and relaxation. Create a restful environment, and don't underestimate the power of a midday nap or a quiet moment of reflection.

4. **Find Purpose and Passion**: Discover what gives you a sense of meaning and fulfillment. Purpose is a powerful driver of longevity, keeping you mentally and emotionally engaged throughout life.

5. **Nurture Relationships and Build Community**: Surround yourself with people who uplift and support you. Cultivate strong social connections, and invest in the relationships that matter most.

The Journey Ahead

Living to 100 may seem like a lofty goal, but by adopting the habits of the world's healthiest and longest-living people, you can set yourself on the path to a vibrant, fulfilling life. Each small change you make—whether in your diet, your movement, or your relationships—brings you one step closer to that goal.

The journey to 100 is not just about adding years to your life but adding life to your years. By prioritizing health, happiness, and connection, you can live a life that is not only long but rich in purpose, joy, and vitality. Here's to a long, healthy, and fulfilling journey ahead!